Mediterranean Seafood & Mushroom Cookbook

50 Delicious Recipes For Your Daily Mediterranean Meals

Alex Brawn

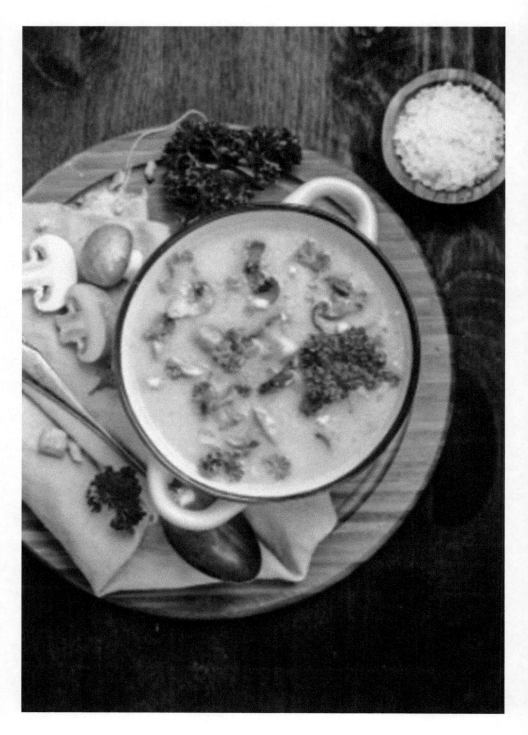

By reading this document, the reader agrees that under no circumstances is the author responsible for any losses, direct or indirect, which are incurred as a result of the use of information contained within this document, including, but not limited to, — errors, omissions, or inaccuracies.

Table of Contents

Pesto mussel and toast

Ingredients

- 160g of fresh or frozen peas
- 70g of pesto
- 500g of mussels, scrubbed, debarred
- 2 thick slices of whole meal bread
- 2 sprigs of fresh basil
- 200g of baby courgettes
- 200g of ripe mixed-color cherry tomatoes
- 50ml of white wine

Directions

- Heat a large pan on a medium-high heat.
- Toast the bread as the pan heats up.
- Remove the toast and spread one quarter of the pesto on each slice of courgrette and tomatoes.
- Raise the heat, place in the mussels.
- Stir in the remaining pesto, courgettes, tomatoes, and peas.
- Add the wine and steam for 4 minutes, shaking the pan occasionally.

- Serve and enjoy.

8

Roasted razor clams

Ingredients

- 2 fresh red chilies
- 2 lemons
- Olive oil
- 3 cloves of garlic
- 3 sprigs of fresh rosemary
- 1kg of razor clams

Directions

- Preheat the oven to oven to high.
- Spread the clams in a roasting tray.
- Spread the sliced chilies, garlic, rosemary, and drizzle with olive oil.
- Let roast for 6 minutes.
- Remove and add lemon juice.
- Drizzle with extra virgin olive oil and serve with crusty bread.
- Enjoy.

Fried clams with rice noodles

Ingredients

- 3 kaffir lime leaves
- 1 kg clams
- 2 teaspoons of fish sauce
- 220g of rice noodles
- 5cm piece of galangal
- 2 limes
- 1 shallot
- 6 red chilies
- 1 tablespoon of rice vinegar
- ½ a bunch of fresh coriander
- Olive oil
- 2 tablespoons red chili paste

Directions

- Cook the noodles as per package Directions. Drain and set aside.
- Combine the clams and noodles in a saucepan over a medium heat.

- Add fry the chili paste briefly, add the galangal, chilies, shallots, and coriander until the shallots soften.
- Add the clams and lime leaves, fry briefly then add the vinegar with bit of water.
- Let cook over a high heat for 2 to 3 minutes covered until all the clams have opened.
- Remove and stir in the noodles, clams, fish sauce, and the juice from 1 lime.
- Let sit for a couple of minutes.
- Serve and enjoy with lime wedges.

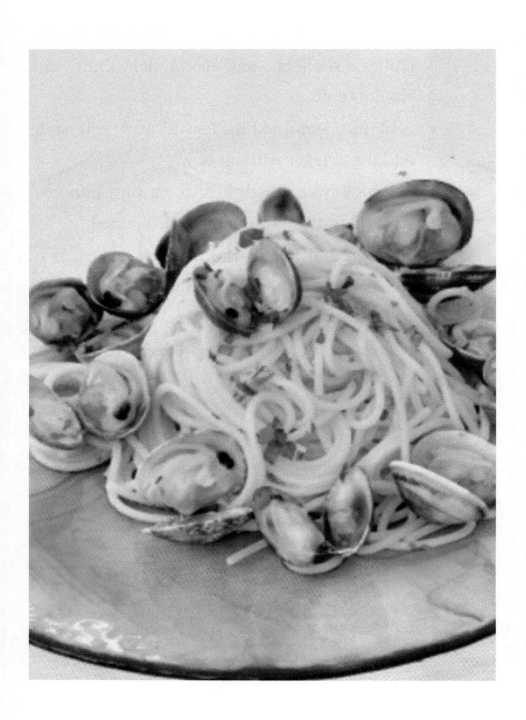

Potted crab with asparagus

Ingredients

- 1 good pinch of ground mace
- 1 fresh red chili
- 225g of unsalted butter
- Sprigs of fresh dill
- 300g of fresh crabmeat
- 1 good pinch of ground cayenne
- 1 whole nutmeg
- 1 Sicilian lemon

Directions

- In a bowl, mix the crab together with the mace, cayenne and nutmeg, lemon zest and juice, chili, and a pinch of sea salt, mix in 125g of the butter.
- Spoon into a small serving bowl, smoothing the surface.
- Scatter with the dill over the top.
- Melt the remaining butter, spoon the clarified butter over the crab.
- Cover and refrigerate for 10 hours until set.

- Serve and enjoy with hot sourdough toasts.

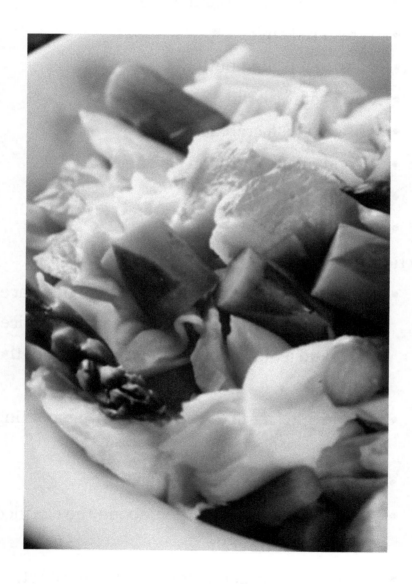

Oyster Rockefeller

Ingredients

- Drops of Tabasco
- 1 small handful of stale breadcrumbs
- 500g of rock salt
- 1 tablespoon of butter
- 3 spring onions
- 6 oysters in deep shells
- 1 stick of celery
- Sprigs of fresh tarragon

Directions

- Place the shells with oyster on a bed of rock salt in baking tray.
- Place spring onions and celery in a food processor with tarragon leaves, and the remaining ingredients.
- Blend to a paste.
- Season, then spoon a little on top of each oyster.
- Cook under a hot grill for 10 minutes.
- Serve and enjoy.

Sticky sesame prawns

The sticky sesame prawns feature great flavors from ginger, garlic, chili, miso, and spring onions perfect for a Mediterranean Sea diet.

Ingredients

- 3 cloves of garlic
- 200ml of fresh cloudy apple juice
- 1 bunch of fresh coriander
- 100g of snow peas
- 2 tablespoons of runny honey
- 200g of tender stem broccoli
- 300g of fine rice noodles
- 3 limes
- 2 carrots
- 1 tablespoon of sweet miso
- 2 tablespoons of sesame seeds
- Vegetable oil
- 16 large raw shell-on green banana king prawns
- 2 spring onions
- ½ of a cucumber

- 1 fresh red chili

- 5cm piece of ginger

- 2 spring onions

- 2 tablespoons of hot chili sauce

Directions

- Place the ginger, garlic, apple juice, miso, honey, and chili sauce and onions in a medium pan. Let boil.

- Lower the heat, let simmer for 5 minutes.

- Cook the rice noodles according to the packet Directions.

- Add the broccoli to blanch with the rice noodles. Drain and toss in sauce and the juice of 2 limes.

- Toast the sesame seeds in a small pan over a medium heat for 3 minutes.

- Heat a splash of olive oil, add the whole prawns and stir-fry for 3 minutes.

- Pour in the remaining sauce, let cook for a further 2 minutes.

- Serve and enjoy with lime wedges.

Spring ahi with new potatoes, dill sauce, yogurt, and chive blossoms

Ingredients

- 8 ounces of ahi
- 1 teaspoon of fennel seeds
- ½ cup of water
- 2 tablespoons of coconut
- ½ teaspoon of kosher salt
- ¼ cup of light olive oil
- 2 ounces of baby spinach
- 1 ounce of dill
- 8 ounces of baby potatoes
- 1 scallion, chopped
- ¼ teaspoon of kosher salt
- 2 teaspoons of lemon juice
- ½ teaspoon of black pepper
- 1 tablespoon of coriander seeds

Directions

- Place potatoes in a small pot , boil over high heat.
- Simmer until fork tender for 25 minutes.

- Blend water, <u>olive oil</u> and spinach.
- Add dill with scallion, <u>salt</u> and pepper and blend until smooth.
- Taste, and adjust.
- Place seeds, <u>salt</u> and pepper on a small plate and mix well.
- Coat ahi with the seed mixture.
- Heat oil over medium high heat.
- Fry for 2 minutes, until golden brown crust.
- Turn over, and cook for 1 minute.
- Serve and enjoy.

Outlaw seafood burger

Ingredients

- 50g of fresh English wasabi
- Pickled onions
- 2 cloves of garlic
- 300ml of sunflower oil
- 1 fresh green chili
- olive oil
- 200g of cod fillet, skinned and pin-boned
- 100g of fresh white and brown crabmeat
- 1 small handful of rocket
- 100g of raw king prawns
- 2 baby gem lettuces
- 4 burger buns
- 2 shallots
- 2 free-range egg yolks
- 1 lemon

Directions

- Heat 2 tablespoons of olive oil over a medium-low heat.

- Add the shallots, garlic, and chili let cook until softened.
- Blend the cod, scoop into a bowl, with crabmeat, stir to combine.
- Add the prawns to the bowl of shallot mixture. Season.
- Mold the mixture into patties.
- Refrigerate for 45 minutes.
- Whisk the egg yolks and lemon juice into a bowl with sunflower oil.
- Stir in the wasabi until combined, season with a pinch of sea salt. Stir in the rocket, refrigerate.
- Thread the lettuces onto a large barbecue skewer.
- Brush the seafood patties with a little oil and barbecue for 3 minutes.
- Toast the burger buns briefly.
- Serve and enjoy.

Japanese inspired Mediterranean Seafood salad

Ingredients

- 1 squid, cleaned
- Olive oil
- ½ tablespoon of soy sauce
- 250g of cooked octopus
- 8 large cooked peeled prawns
- 1 handful of salad leaves
- 1 small handful of edible flowers
- 1 tablespoon of sesame seeds
- 3 tablespoons of toasted sesame oil
- 1 tablespoon yuzu juice
- 1 teaspoon of togarashi spice mix

Directions

- Heat ½ tablespoon of olive oil over a medium heat.
- Cook the squid for 4 minutes.
- Add soy sauce over high heat, stir continuously for 2 minutes.
- Transfer to a salad bowl.

- Toast the sesame seeds in a dry frying pan until golden, combine with sesame seeds, sesame oil, yuzu juice, and togarashi spice mix.
- Place sliced octopus with prawns in the salad bowl.
- Serve and enjoy with edible flowers.

Prawn and chorizo orzo

Ingredients

- 400ml of passata
- 400g of large cooked peeled king prawns
- 200g of quality chorizo
- 200g of cherry tomatoes
- 300g of orzo
- ½ a bunch of fresh basil
- 4 tablespoons of olive oil
- 2 cloves of garlic
- 2 tablespoons of sherry vinegar

Directions

- Preheat the oven to 350°F.
- Heat half of olive oil, fry the garlic with chorizo for 3 minutes.
- Deglaze the pan with the vinegar.
- Add the passata with orzo and water boil, lower heat let simmer 15 minutes, stirring occasionally.
- Spread the cherry tomatoes over a baking tray, drizzled with the rest of the olive oil, season.

- Roast for until soft.
- Stir half the basil into the pasta, along with the prawns.
- Serve and enjoy.

Prawns with fennel

Ingredients

- 10 large raw prawns
- Sprigs of fresh flat-leaf parsley
- Olive oil
- 750g of ripe cherry tomatoes
- 1 lemon
- 1 bulb of fennel
- 1 large wineglass of white wine
- 2 cloves of garlic

Directions

- Heat olive oil and fry the garlic till golden.
- Add the fennel and parsley stalks, sauté for 10 minutes over low heat.
- Add tomatoes to the pan with the wine, let boil and simmer for 10 minutes.
- Add prawns to the pan, let cook for 4 minutes or until cooked and pink.
- Stir through parsley leaves and season.
- Serve and enjoy with lemon wedges.

262. Love dumplings

Ingredients

- Sprigs of fresh basil
- Sprigs of fresh mint
- 1 lime
- 1 large shallot
- 4 tablespoons of fish sauce
- 2 cloves of garlic
- 4 spring onions
- ½ a bunch of fresh coriander
- 200g of raw peeled prawns
- 4 tablespoons of caster sugar
- 16 round dumpling wrappers
- 1 fresh red chili
- 100g of glass noodles
- Chili sauce
- 1 tablespoon of unsalted peanuts
- 1 lettuce

Directions

- Combine chili, lime juice, sugar, fish sauce, and water.

- Dunk in a cute bowl, save the rest for dressing lettuce, herb and noodle salad.
- Place the prawns together with the shallot, garlic, coriander, and the whites of the spring onions in a bowl.
- Season with black pepper and a pinch of sea salt, mix.
- Lay out your wrappers and spoon a teaspoon of filling into the middle of each.
- Brush the edges of one wrapper with water, fold in half, then pleat and pinch the edges together to secure. Repeat for the rest.
- Place an oiled pan over a medium heat.
- Add the dumplings with a splash of water, and cover for 3 minutes.
- Cook noodles according to the packet Directions.
- Toast, and crush the peanuts.
- Serve and enjoy.

Mushroom cannelloni

Ingredients

- 250g of dried cannelloni tubes
- 120g of Cheddar cheese
- 2 cloves of garlic
- 2 leeks
- 1-liter semi-skimmed milk
- 2 small onions
- 750g of shell nut mushrooms
- 75g of plain flour
- Olive oil

Directions

- Preheat your oven ready to 350°F.
- Pulse the onions with garlic in a food processor.
- Add into a large casserole pan on a medium-high heat with olive oil.
- Add pulsed leeks with mushroom, stir into the pan.
- Let cook for 15 minutes, stirring regularly.
- Season to perfection.

- Pour 3 tablespoons of olive oil into another different pan over a medium heat.
- Whisk in the flour and milk, let simmer for 5 minutes, add cheese and season.
- Pour 1/3 of the sauce into roasting tray.
- Push both ends of each pasta tube into it to fill, lining them up in the tray.
- Pour over the rest of the sauce, slice the reserved mushrooms for decoration.
- Drizzle with olive oil.
- Let bake for 45 minutes.
- Serve and enjoy.

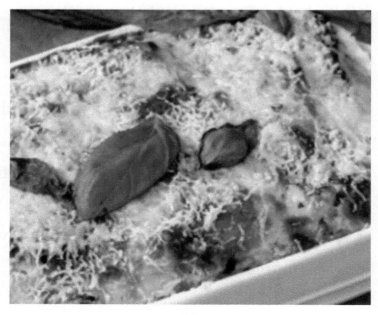

Mushroom stroganoff

Ingredients

- 1 tablespoon of baby capers
- 50ml of whisky
- 1 red onion
- 2 cloves of garlic
- 80g of half-fat crème fraiche
- Smoked paprika
- 4 silver skin pickled onions
- 2 cornichons
- 400g of mixed mushrooms
- 4 sprigs of fresh flat-leaf parsley
- Olive oil

Directions

- Place a large non-stick frying pan over a high heat.
- Place in the mushrooms together with the red onions, shake into one layer, dry-fry for 5 minutes, stirring regularly.
- Drizzle in olive oil.

- Add the garlic together with the pickled onions, parsley stalks, cornichons, and capers.
- Shortly, pour in the whisky, tilt the pan to flame,
- Then, add ¼ of a teaspoon of paprika together with the crème fraiche and parsley, toss.
- Season with sea salt and black pepper.
- Divide between plates, sprinkle over a little paprika.
- Serve and enjoy with fluffy rice.

Mushroom toad in the hole

Ingredients

- Red wine vinegar
- 4 free-range large eggs
- 4 sprigs of rosemary
- 175g of plain flour
- 2 cloves of garlic
- 175ml of whole milk
- 4 large Portobello mushrooms
- 2 onions
- 250ml of smooth porter
- Olive oil

Directions

- Preheat your oven to 400°F.
- Whisk the eggs with flour, a pinch of sea salt, milk, and bit of water into a smooth batter.
- Place the mushrooms cap side down in a large non-stick roasting tray.
- Drizzle with olive oil.
- Season with salt and black pepper.
- Let roast for 30 minutes.

- Place onions and sliced mushroom peelings, some rosemary in a pan on a medium-low heat with bit of olive oil.
- Let cook for 15 minutes, stirring occasionally.
- Add the porter with red wine vinegar, stir in the remaining flour shortly.
- Season, add garlic, remaining rosemary, drizzle, rub with a little olive oil.
- Remove the tray, pour the batter into the tray, place mushrooms close to the center.
- Sprinkle over the oiled garlic and rosemary.
- Place in oven for 25 minutes.
- Serve and enjoy with gravy.

Wild mushroom and venison stroganoff

Ingredients

- 1 knob of butter
- 1 onion
- 1 clove of garlic
- Extra virgin olive oil
- 150ml of soured cream
- 250g of mixed wild mushrooms
- 1 lemon
- 1 teaspoon of sweet paprika
- 150g of basmati rice
- ½ a bunch of fresh flat-leaf parsley
- 1 handful of cornichons
- 300g of venison saddle
- Gin

Directions

- Cook the rice per the package Directions, until just undercooked.
- Drain any excess water. Steam covered till ready.

- Place the onion and garlic with olive oil into a large frying pan over a medium heat, cook for 5 minutes.
- Stir the paprika into the pan with the mushrooms, let cook for 5 minutes.
- Season the venison with sea salt and black pepper.
- Fry meat for 1 minute.
- Add and flame the gin, stir in the butter with gratings of lemon zest and lemon juice.
- Stir in most of the soured cream, season, let simmer for 1 minute.
- Swirl through the remaining soured cream, scatter over the sliced cornichons and parsley.
- Sprinkle with a pinch of paprika.
- Serve and enjoy immediately.

Crispy mushroom shawarma

Ingredients

- 4 tablespoons of tahini
- 800g of Portobello and oyster mushrooms
- 1 red onion
- 2 tablespoons of dukkha
- 2 cloves of garlic
- 1 teaspoon of ground allspice
- Olive oil
- 2 tablespoons of pomegranate molasses
- 200g of natural yoghurt
- 10 radishes
- 1 teaspoon of ground cumin
- ½ cucumber
- 100g of ripe cherry tomatoes
- 1 tablespoon white wine vinegar
- 2 preserved lemons
- 1 teaspoon of smoked paprika
- 200g jar of pickled jalapeño chilies
- 1 bunch of fresh mint
- 4 large flatbreads

Directions

- Sieve yogurt into a bowl.
- Place Portobello mushrooms, onion, garlic, and lemons, and bash in a mortar with olive oil, black pepper, and allspices.
- Muddle and toss with all the mushrooms and onions, let marinate overnight.
- Preheat the oven to /475°F.
- Place mushrooms and onions on a large baking tray, roast for 20 minutes, turning occasionally.
- Drizzle over the pomegranate molasses for the last 3 minutes.
- Toss the cucumber, radishes, and tomatoes with a pinch of salt and the vinegar.
- Combine jalapeños and mint leaves, bend until fine.
- Pour back into the jar
- Warm the flatbreads, spread with tahini, sprinkle with pickled vegetables, remaining mint leaves and dukkha.

- Carve and scatter over the gnarly vegetables, dollop over yoghurt.
- Roll up, slice and enjoy.

Pithivier pie

Ingredients

- Olive oil
- 800ml of semi-skimmed milk
- 2 x 320g sheets of all-butter puff pastry
- 1 large free-range egg
- 2 large leeks
- 1 knob of unsalted butter
- 2 cloves of garlic
- 1 bunch of fresh flat-leaf parsley
- 400g of mixed mushrooms
- 75g of plain flour
- 120g of blue cheese
- 2 teaspoons of English mustard
- 1 whole celeriac

Directions

- Preheat the oven to 400°F.
- Roast the celeriac for 1 hour and 30 minutes.
- Slice and season with sea salt and black pepper.

- Place leeks, mushroom, garlic, and butter in a large casserole pan on a medium heat, cook for 15 minutes.
- Stir in the flour, mustard, milk, let simmer for 5 minutes, stirring regularly.
- Stir in the parsley, crumble in the cheese, season when off heat.
- Line bowl with Clingfilm.
- Arrange slices of celeriac in and around the bowl until covered, layer with the remaining celeriac in the bowl, finishing with celeriac.
- Pull over the Clingfilm, weigh it down, refrigerate overnight with the remaining sauce.
- Preheat the oven to 350°F.
- On greaseproof paper, roll both sheets of pastry out to around.
- Unwrap the filling parcel and place in the middle of one sheet.
- Beat the egg and brush around the edge of the pastry and celeriac.

- Lay the second piece of pastry on top, smoothing around the shape of the filling, seal.
- Bake at the bottom of the oven for 2 hours.
- Serve an enjoy.

Midnight pan-cooked breakfast

Ingredients

- Crusty bread
- Sausages
- Mushrooms
- Olive oil
- Higher-welfare smoked
- Ripe tomatoes
- Large free-range eggs

Directions

- Preheat your pan to high heat.
- Place sausages in the pan at one side.
- Place a pile of mushrooms over the pan with olive oil.
- Coat the mushrooms with oil, season with sea salt and black pepper.
- Push to one side, then lay some slices of bacon and halved tomatoes in the pan.
- Cook for briefly until the bacon is crisp, flip the bacon over.

- Add 3 eggs at different ends of the pan dribbling around the sausages, bacon, tomatoes and mushrooms.
- Lower the heat, continue to cook for 1 minute.
- Serve and enjoy.

Garlic mushroom pasta

Ingredients

- 2 cloves of garlic
- 2 heaped tablespoons of half-fat crème fraiche
- 250g of mixed mushrooms
- 150g of dried toffee
- 25g of Parmesan cheese

Directions

- Cook the pasta in a pan of boiling salted water per the package Directions.
- Drain and reserve some cooking water for later.
- Place garlic, olive oil, mushrooms in a large non-stick frying pan on a medium.
- Season with sea salt and black pepper, let cook for 8 minutes, tossing regularly.
- Toss the drained pasta into the mushroom pan with a splash of reserved cooking water.
- Add grated Parmesan with crème fraiche.
- Taste, and adjust the seasoning.
- Serve and enjoy.

Baked garlicky mushrooms

Ingredients

- 40g of Cheddar cheese
- 4 cloves of garlic
- 350g of ripped mixed-color cherry tomatoes
- 4 large Portobello mushrooms
- ½ a bunch of fresh sage

Directions

- Preheat the oven to 400°F.
- Place mushrooms in a roasting tray, drizzle with olive oil and red wine vinegar.
- Add a pinch of sea salt and black pepper and toss.
- Place in garlic and sage leaves, sit the mushrooms stalk side up on the top.
- Let bake for 10 minutes.
- Remove the tray, crumble the cheese into the mushroom cups and sprinkle over the reserved garlic and sage.
- Return to the oven for 15 more minutes.
- Serve and enjoy.

Mushroom bourguignon

Ingredients

- 500ml of red wine
- 6 sprigs of fresh thyme
- 12 shallots
- 25g of dried porcini mushrooms
- 4 Portobello mushrooms
- 2 fresh bay leaves
- 2 large carrots
- 1 tablespoon of tomato purée
- 120g of shiitake mushrooms
- 2 cloves of garlic
- 200g of shell nut mushrooms
- 25g of unsalted butter
- Olive oil

Directions

- Heat half of the butter with olive oil in a casserole pan over a medium heat.
- Fry all the mushrooms in batches, until colored.

- Heat the remaining butter in the pan, fry shallots with carrots, and garlic for 8 minutes, stirring occasionally.
- Add the thyme together with the bay and wine.
- Strain in the porcini liquid with porcini and tomato puree into the pan let simmer for 25 minutes or until the wine has reduced slightly.
- Season to taste and remove the thyme stalks and bay leaves.
- Stir in the cooked mushrooms into the sauce with any juices, heating through briefly.
- Serve and enjoy with creamy mash on the side.

Mushroom and lentil pappardelle Bolognese

Ingredients

- 1 x 400g tin of plum tomatoes
- 2 cloves of garlic
- 1 stick of celery
- Parmesan cheese
- Olive oil
- 2 fresh bay leaves
- ½ a bunch of fresh thyme
- 4 large Portobello mushrooms
- 1 carrot
- ½ a bunch of fresh baby basil
- 100g of dried Puy lentils
- 2 tablespoons of tomato purée
- 1 onion
- 400ml of organic vegetable stock
- 350 g dried pappardelle

Directions

- Blend carrot together with the onion, celery, and garlic in a food processor, until finely chopped.
- Heat splash of olive oil over a medium heat.
- Add the chopped vegetable mixture together with bay leaves and thyme leaves, let cook for 10 minutes, stirring until soft.
- Chop mushrooms in the food processor.
- Add to the pan, cook for 3 minutes.
- Stir in the lentils together with the tomato purée and stock, squish in the plum tomatoes.
- Season, lower the heat, let cook, stirring occasionally, for 30 minutes covered.
- Cook the pappardelle according to package Directions.
- Drain any excess water, stir it through the Bolognese sauce.
- Sprinkle over with basil leaves and grating of Parmesan.
- Serve and enjoy.

Mushroom curry

The mushroom curry is a perfect choice of Mediterranean Sea diet. It is packed with flavors and a meatless vegetable source.

Ingredients

- 1 bunch of fresh coriander
- 1 heaped teaspoon of medium curry powder
- 500g of mixed mushrooms
- 400g of brown basmati rice
- 2 cloves of garlic
- 1 x 400ml tin of light coconut milk
- 5cm piece of ginger
- 1 onion
- 1 fresh red chili
- 500g of ripped mixed-color tomatoes
- Groundnut oil
- 1 tablespoon of mango chutney
- 1 teaspoon of turmeric
- 1 teaspoon of fenugreek
- 2 limes
- 1 heaped teaspoon of black mustard seeds

- 30g of paneer

Directions

- Preheat your oven ready to 400°F.
- Toast the mushrooms over the hob over a medium heat for 8 minutes, until nutty and golden.
- Add garlic, ginger, onion, chili, and olive oil with spices, toss until the spices are toasted, stirring continuously.
- Add the tomatoes together with the mango chutney and coconut milk, stir.
- Season with sea salt and black pepper.
- Top with bits of the paneer and place in the oven.
- Let cook for 30 minutes, or until gnarly.
- Then, cook the rice as instructed on the package.
- Taste, and adjust the seasoning accordingly.
- Spoon the curry over the rice, spread with coriander leaves.
- Serve and enjoy.

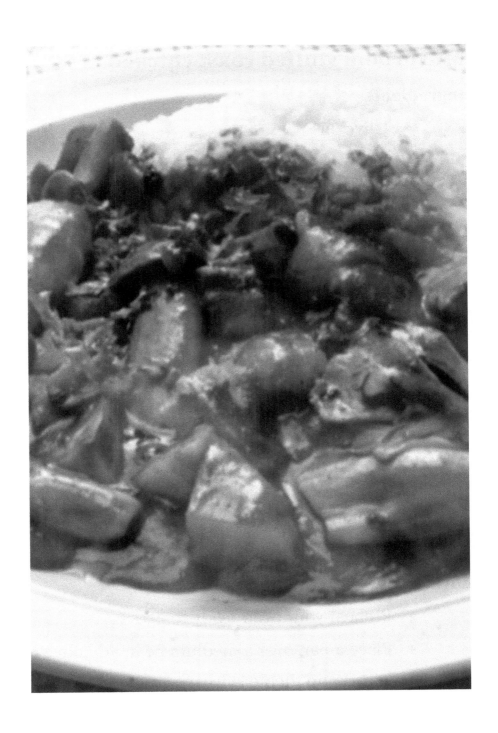

Mushroom stuffed roast chicken

Ingredients

- Olive oil
- 2 cloves of garlic
- 1 bunch of fresh thyme
- 1.2kg of whole free-range chicken
- 200g of button, brown, shell nut
- 1 large bulb of fennel
- 80g of unsalted butter
- 10g of mixed dried mushrooms
- 150ml of white wine
- 1 bunch of fresh flat-leaf parsley
- 1 handful of ripe cherry tomatoes
- Truffle oil
- 1 onion
- 2 sticks of celery

Directions

- Preheat your oven ready to 350°F.
- Place a pan over a medium heat, add olive oil, garlic, and thyme leaves.

- Tear in both fresh and rehydrated mushrooms with the soaking liquid.
- Let cook for 20 minutes, stirring continuously.
- Remove, roughly chop on a board. Shift to a bowl.
- Add butter to the mushroom mix.
- Stir parsley leaves through the mushrooms, with truffle oil and a pinch of sea salt and black pepper.
- Add celery, onion, tomatoes, wine, and fennel to a large roasting tray.
- Stuff the mushroom filling into the chicken.
- Place the chicken in the tray on top of the vegetables and drizzle with olive oil, season.
- Let roast for 2 hours.
- Let rest for 10 minutes.
- Serve and enjoy with seasonal steamed greens and roasted potatoes.

Grilled mushroom and peppers

Ingredients

- Olive oil
- 1 lemon
- 130ml of fat-free plain yoghurt
- 2 red peppers
- 50g of feta cheese
- 6 sprigs of fresh flat-leaf parsley
- 100g of spring onions
- Extra virgin olive oil
- 4 large field mushrooms
- 200g of brown rice
- 10g of shelled pistachios

Directions

- Cook rice in salted boiling water for 25 minutes.
- Drain any excess water, set aside for later.
- Add half of the lemon juice into a small bowl.
- Add the yoghurt, season with sea salt and black pepper.

- Steam black pepper for around 10 minutes, let cool.
- Drizzle olive oil over the mushrooms, season with salt and pepper.
- Toast pistachios in a large pan, roughly chop.
- Reduce heat to medium, then return the pan to the heat.
- Place the mushrooms into the hot pan, cook for 5 minutes covered.
- Stir the parsley, olive oil, pinch of pepper and spring onions through the cooked rice.
- Sprinkle in the lemon zest and squeeze over the remaining juice.
- Pile the herby rice onto plates. slice and toss the mushrooms with the peppers and resting juices.
- Serve and enjoy lemony yogurt.

Mushroom and cauliflower penne

Mushroom and cauliflower penne is insanely packed with vegetables and herbs for a great Mediterranean Sea diet. Above and beyond, cauliflower is a great source of vitamin C.

Ingredients

- 100g of ricotta cheese
- 2 cloves of garlic
- 1 lemon
- 1 onion
- 1 fresh red chili
- 15g of fresh thyme
- 20g of Parmesan cheese
- 320g of cauliflower
- Olive oil
- 250g of shell nut mushrooms
- 200g of whole wheat penne
- 15g of fresh flat-leaf parsley

Directions

- Heat olive oil over a medium heat.

- Add the garlic together with the onion, chili, and thyme, cook for 10 minutes.
- Add the sliced mushrooms and cauliflower, cook for 10 minutes when covered.
- Cook pasta as instructed on the package. Drain any excess water, reserving some.
- Mash the cauliflower mixture.
- Stir in the ricotta.
- Season with sea salt, black pepper, and lemon juice.
- Return the pasta to the pan, off the heat.
- Place in the sauce and stir well, adding splashes of the cooking water to loosen.
- Taste, and season with salt, pepper and the remaining lemon juice.
- Stir in the sliced raw mushrooms, Parmesan cheese, and parsley leaves.
- Serve and enjoy.

Asparagus with mushroom mayonnaise

Ingredients

- 200g of button mushrooms
- 16 asparagus spears
- ½ tablespoon of balsamic vinegar
- 25g of broad beans
- 40g of mayonnaise
- 40g of cheddar cheese
- 1 tablespoon of truffle oil
- 1 handful of watercress

Directions

- Blitz the mushrooms together with the vinegar and sea salt in a food processor until combined.
- Spoon the mixture into a cheesecloth and leave it overnight to strain the liquid.
- Preheat a griddle pan over a high heat.
- Cook the asparagus spears for 3 minutes, turn and cook for 2 minutes.
- Divide broad beans between four plates with the asparagus.

- Grate the cheese over, drizzle with the olive oil.
- Serve and enjoy with the salad leaves and mushroom mayonnaise.

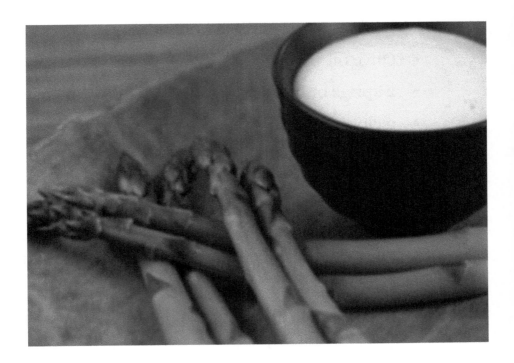

Mushroom sourdough bruschetta

Ingredients

- 200g of mixed wild mushrooms
- 2 Portobello mushrooms
- 2 slices of sourdough bread
- 2 tablespoons of fresh hollandaise
- Olive oil
- 2 sprigs of fresh tarragon
- 2 cloves of garlic
- 20g of unsalted butter

Directions

- Start by preheating your oven to 400°F.
- Place the Portobello mushrooms on a baking tray.
- Drizzle with bit of olive oil and spread with crush garlic and dot on half of the butter.
- Let roast in the oven for 10 minutes.
- Heat a griddle pan over a high heat and chargrill the bread until golden grill-mark lines appear.

- Add torn wild mushrooms, garlic and butter to a frying pan over a medium-high heat.
- Fry until the mushrooms are cooked. Stir the hollandaise through.
- Top each toast with a roasted Portobello and a spoonful of the wild mushrooms.
- Serve and enjoy.

Garlic mushroom burgers

Ingredients

- 1 lemon
- 2 cloves of garlic
- 2 sprigs of fresh flat-leaf parsley
- 1 handful of rocket
- 2 burger buns or ciabatta
- 35g of butter
- 2 large mushrooms
- English mustard

Directions

- Preheat your oven ready to 400°F.
- Combine the garlic and parsley leaves with the softened butter.
- Fill up the mushrooms with the butter.
- Wrap in tin foil and bake in the oven for 15 minutes, or till the mushrooms are cooked.
- Split the burger buns or ciabatta.
- Unwrap the mushrooms and pour the juices onto the bread.

- Smear with mustard and top with a mushroom.
- Serve and enjoy.

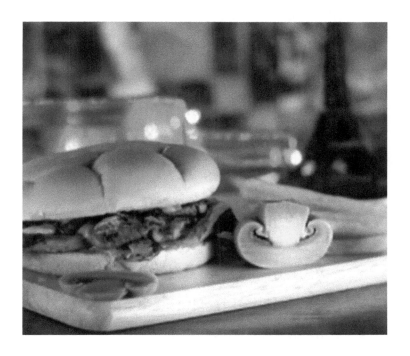

Mushroom and Tunworth cheese pies

Ingredients

- 2 heaped teaspoons of English mustard
- 1 handful of porcini mushrooms
- Plain flour
- 120g of Tunworth cheese
- 1kg of fresh mixed mushrooms
- 500g of all-butter puff pastry
- 4 cloves of garlic
- 2 onions
- ½ a bunch of fresh thyme
- 1 tablespoon of Worcestershire sauce
- 300g of potatoes
- Olive oil
- 1 large knob of butter
- 500ml of organic vegetable stock
- ½ a bunch of fresh flat-leaf parsley
- 1 large free-range egg

Directions

- Heat olive oil and fry the garlic with thyme leaves, and butter over a medium heat until lightly golden.
- Add the onions, let sauté for 10 minutes.
- Add and fry the fresh mushrooms for 5 minutes.
- Add soaked porcini to the pan, let fry for 4 minutes.
- Add and season the stock and potatoes.
- Bring to the boil, let simmer for 30 minutes over low heat.
- Stir in the parsley.
- Divide the filling between small pie dishes, reserving some for later.
- Scatter Tunworth into each of the pie dishes.
- Preheat the oven to 400°F.
- Beat the egg and brush it over the pies, bake oven for 20 minutes.
- In a pan, stir the mustard and Worcestershire sauce into the remaining filling.

- Serve and enjoy with a dollop of English mustard.

Super noodle ramen with kale and barbecue mushrooms

Ingredients

- 400g of mixed mushrooms
- Olive oil
- 1 large bunch of kale
- 2 tablespoons of dark miso paste
- 4 tablespoons of sesame seeds
- 1 bulb garlic
- 2 tablespoons of white miso paste
- 4 tablespoons of teriyaki sauce
- 1 heaped teaspoon of tahini
- 1 tablespoon of low-salt soy sauce
- 250g of brown-rice ramen noodles
- 2 tablespoons mirin
- 1 fresh red chili
- 1 large brown onion
- 1 tablespoon of sugar
- 1 tablespoon of white wine vinegar

Directions

- Heat a splash of olive oil over a medium heat.

- Cook the whole garlic and sliced onion for 30 minutes
- Add water to the pan. Boil, then simmer for 20 minutes.
- Preheat the oven to 200°F.
- Roast kale leaves for 30 minutes.
- Drain, squash onion and garlic.
- In a small bowl, mix both miso pastes and the tahini with some broth.
- Stir this back into the main pan and season with soy sauce and mirin.
- Place kale in the bowl, scrunch with the sugar, vinegar, and a pinch of sea salt, slice and toss the red chili.
- Dry-fry the mushrooms for 10 minutes.
- Pour in the teriyaki and a splash of oil and keep them all moving around the pan for 6 to 8 minutes.
- Cook the noodles in the broth as instructed on the package.
- Toast the sesame seeds in a dry frying pan.
- Serve and enjoy sprinkled with toasted seeds.

Mixed mushroom stuffing

Ingredients

- 25g of dried porcini
- 4 cloves of garlic
- 350g of mixed wild mushrooms
- 80ml of olive oil
- 400g of closed cup or shell nut mushrooms
- ½ a bunch of fresh thyme
- 1 bunch of fresh flat-leaf parsley
- 2 fresh bay leaves
- 350g of stale bread
- 2 shallots
- 100g of pecans or hazelnuts

Directions

- Heat the olive oil, add the shallot together with garlic.
- Cook over a medium heat for 8 minutes, stirring occasionally.
- Add porcini, mushroom, bay, and thyme leaves until the mushrooms are well softened.
- Preheat the oven to 375°F.

- Add the chunks of bread with a pinch of sea salt and black pepper, pecans, and bit of porcini's reserved soaking liquid. Combine well.

- Add most of the parsley and stir it through then tip the stuffing into a lightly greased baking dish cover with foil.

- Bake for 35 minutes, remove the foil, let cook for more 10 minutes.

- Serve and enjoy.

Creamy mushroom vol-au-vents

Ingredients

- ½ lemon
- 350g of all butter puff pastry
- Plain flour
- Sprigs of fresh flat-leaf parsley
- 1 free-range egg
- 2 cloves of garlic
- 2 tablespoons of crème fraiche
- 1 dried red chili
- 250g of mixed mushrooms
- Olive oil

Directions

- Preheat your oven ready to 300°F.
- Align a baking tray with greaseproof paper.
- Roll out the pastry on a lightly floured surface, cut out 12 rounds.
- Place the circles on the baking tray and prick their centers severally.
- Beat the egg, then egg wash the circles.
- Bake for about 12 minutes until puffed up.

- Heat a lug of oil in a large pan.
- Then, cook the mushrooms together with the garlic and chili, until golden.
- Squeeze in the lemon juice, add crème fraiche.
- Season, fold through the parsley.
- Cut holes and fill with the creamy mushrooms.
- Serve and enjoy.

Super tasty miso broth

Ingredients

- 1 red onion
- Groundnut oil
- 150g of mixed exotic mushrooms
- 1 x 5cm piece of ginger
- 1 heaped teaspoon of miso paste
- 800ml of really good chicken stock
- 6 radishes
- Rice or white wine vinegar
- 20g of dried porcini mushrooms
- 1 x 200g of skinless free-range chicken breast
- 150g of mixed brown
- 1 handful of colorful curly kale
- 1 sheet of nori

Directions

- Begin by cooking the rice according to the package Directions.
- Place onions and groundnut oil in a pan over medium heat, cook for a few minutes, stirring occasionally.

- Lower the heat, add the ginger together with the miso paste, porcini, and stock and soaking water, let simmer for 20 minutes.
- Toss radish with vinegar and a small pinch of sea salt.
- Stir in chicken, kale, nori, and mushroom through the broth.
- Re-cover and cook for 4 minutes.
- Drain and divide the rice between your bowls with the radishes.
- Season the broth.
- Serve and enjoy.

Cranberry and pistachio nut toast

Ingredients

- 2 sprigs of fresh thyme
- 1 small handful of dried porcini
- 2 sprigs of fresh rosemary
- 100g of almonds
- 2 tablespoons of soft light brown sugar
- 500ml of hot organic vegetable stock
- 2 sticks of celery
- 1 lemon
- 2 red onions
- 1 handful of sourdough
- 2 cloves of garlic
- olive oil
- 150g of risotto rice or pearl barley
- 100ml of white wine
- 200g of mixed wild mushrooms
- 2 large free-range eggs
- 100g of pistachios
- 125g of vegetarian Cheddar cheese
- 200g of fresh cranberries

- 1 fresh red chili
- 2 sprigs of fresh sage

Directions

- Heat a drizzle of oil over a low heat.
- Add the celery with onion, and garlic, let cook for 10 minutes.
- Add the rice, let cook for a minute, add the wine and stir until absorbed.
- Add chopped porcini to the pan.
- Add the hot stock, stirring to be completely absorbed, in 20 minutes.
- Preheat the oven to 375°F.
- Fry the wild mushrooms in a little oil over a medium heat for 10 minutes.
- Add breadcrumbs together with the Cheddar, lemon zest, chili, eggs and chopped herbs, season, and mix.
- Cook the sugar with the cranberries in a pan over a medium heat for 2 minutes, then tip into the tin and spread evenly.
- Pile on the nut-roast mixture and pack it down.

- Cover with a foil, let bake for 45 minutes, remove the foil, continue to cook for a 15 minutes.
- Serve and enjoy sliced.

Breakfast popovers

Ingredients

- 2 tablespoons of natural yoghurt
- 1 large free-range egg
- 2 heaped tablespoons of cottage cheese
- 15 g Parmesan cheese
- 1 slice of smoked ham
- ½ a lemon
- 1 heaped tablespoon of whole meal self-raising flour
- 1 ripe plum tomato
- 2 shell nut mushrooms
- 2 handfuls of rocket
- Hot chili sauce

Directions

- Place the flour in a bowl and beat well with the egg and cottage cheese.
- Finely chop the ham, tomato and mushrooms, and stir through the mixture with a pinch of sea salt and black pepper.

- Put a large non-stick frying pan on a medium-low heat.
- Place heaped spoonful of the mixture into the pan to give six popovers.
- Leave them to get nicely golden for a few minutes, then flip over and gently flatten to 1cm thick with a palette knife.
- Remove the popovers once golden on every side, then turn the heat off.
- Finely grate the Parmesan into the pan to melt.
- Place the popovers on top, wait for the Parmesan to sizzle.
- Swirl some chili sauce through the yoghurt.
- Toss the rocket in a squeeze of lemon juice.
- Serve and enjoy.

Thai green chicken curry

Ingredients

- 5cm piece of ginger
- 750g of skinless free-range chicken thighs
- 4 green chilies
- Groundnut oil
- 400g of mixed oriental mushrooms
- 2 shallots
- ½ a bunch of fresh Thai basil
- 1 teaspoon of ground cumin
- 1 x 400g tin of light coconut milk
- 1 organic chicken stock cube
- ½ a bunch of fresh coriander
- 200g of mange tout
- 2 limes
- 6 kaffir lime leaves
- 2 tablespoons of fish sauce
- 4 cloves of garlic
- 2 lemongrass stalks

Directions

- Process garlic, shallots, lemongrass, cumin, coriander, fish sauce, and ginger in a food processor.
- Heat 1 tablespoon of olive oil over a medium heat.
- Add the chicken and fry for 7 minutes.
- Return the pan to a medium heat, add the mushrooms, fry for 5 minutes.
- Transfer to a plate using a slotted spoon.
- Add the Thai green paste over low heat, cook for 5 minutes, stirring occasionally.
- Pour in the coconut milk with boiling water.
- Crumble in the stock cube and add the lime leaves.
- Turn the heat up and bring gently to the boil, then simmer for 10 minutes.
- Add the mange tout cook for 2 minutes.
- Season with sea salt and freshly ground black pepper.
- Serve and enjoy.

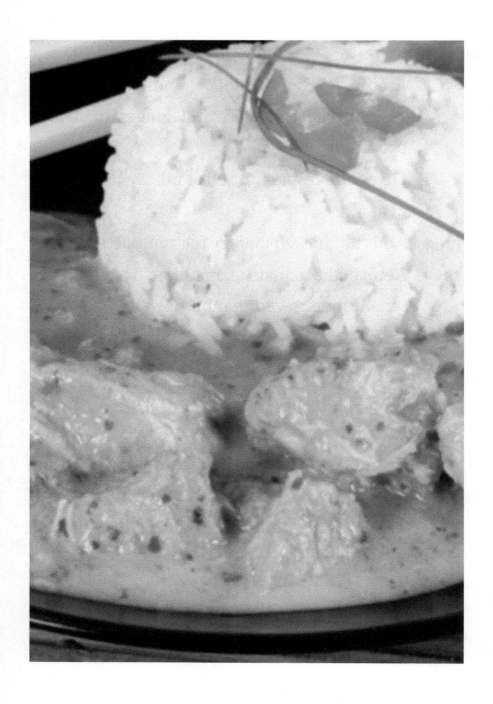

Vegan noodles

Ingredients

- 2 tablespoons low-salt soy sauce
- ½ tablespoon of rice wine
- 300g of mixed oriental mushrooms
- 2 cloves of garlic
- 200g of thin rice noodles
- 1 tablespoon of agave syrup
- 1 fresh red chili
- 100g of baby spinach
- 1 teaspoon of sesame oil
- 5cm of piece of ginger
- 200g of courgettes
- ½ bunch of fresh coriander
- 2 limes
- 6 spring onions
- Groundnut oil
- 1 teaspoon of corn flour

Directions

- Cook the noodles according to packet Directions.

- Drain any excess water. Set aside.
- Heat oil over a high heat, add fry the mushroom for 4 minutes.
- Add the chopped garlic together with the chili, courgette, ginger, coriander stalks, and white part of spring onions. Fry until lightly golden.
- Then combine corn flour with 2 tablespoons of water, mix with soy, agave syrup, sesame oil, and rice wine in a pan.
- Cook for 3 minutes.
- Add chopped spinach with the noodles. Toss, then tear in coriander leaves.
- Serve and enjoy with lime wedges and sambal topping with spring onions.

Vegan mushroom rolls

Ingredients

- 2 sheets of ready-rolled puff pastry
- Olive oil
- 500g of shell nut mushrooms
- 2 cloves of garlic
- 2 teaspoons of sesame seeds
- Almond milk
- 1 tablespoon of Dijon mustard
- 100ml of white wine
- Sea salt
- Freshly ground black pepper
- 1 onion
- 80g of fresh white breadcrumbs
- ½ bunch of fresh flat-leaf parsley
- 2 stalks of celery
- 2 sprigs of fresh thyme

Directions

- Preheat your oven to 400°F.
- Then, line a large baking tray with greaseproof paper.

- Add onion and celery in a heated pan with olive oil over a medium-high heat. Cook for 15 minutes.
- Add crushed garlic with chopped mushrooms, let cook for 5 minutes, or until the mushrooms start to soften.
- Add the mustard and wine.
- Season with salt and pepper.
- Lower the heat, let cook for 10 minutes, or until all the liquid has bubbled away.
- Let cool.
- Add the cooled mushroom mixture and breadcrumbs to a large bowl.
- Add parsley leaves with thyme leaves. Stir well.
- Season to taste.
- Spoon a quarter of the mushroom mixture place on the pastry, mold into a long sausage shape.
- Brush the almond milk along the pastry edges, fold one of the long sides of the pastry up over the filling. Seal.

- Repeat with the remaining ingredients until all are done.
- Place the rolls on the prepared baking tray, brush with the almond milk and sprinkle over the sesame seeds.
- Bake for 25 minutes, or until golden.
- Serve and enjoy.

Mushroom and squash vegetarian wellington

Ingredients

- 25g of sultanas
- 1 small dried red chili, crumbled
- 250g of shell nut mushrooms
- ½ teaspoon of ground cinnamon
- 1 tablespoon of coriander seeds
- 500g of all butter puff pastry
- 1 sprig fresh rosemary
- 50g of pine nuts
- Olive oil
- 2 red onions, peeled and sliced
- Sea salt
- 1 splash milk
- freshly ground black pepper
- 1 small butternut squash
- 1 small bunch fresh sage
- 100g of vac-packed shell nuts
- 2 slices sourdough bread
- 1 free-range egg

- 3 cloves garlic
- 1 lemon
- 20g of butter
- 200g of Swiss chard

Directions

- Preheat the oven to 400°F.
- Add squash wedges to a large roasting tray with a splash of olive oil, chili, cinnamon, coriander seeds, rosemary leaves, bash 2 minutes to coat with the seasoning.
- Cover with tin foil, bake for around 45 minutes, let cool, then tear into bite-sized chunks.
- Add onion in a heated pan with olive oil.
- Season with salt and pepper, cook, stirring occasionally, until softened.
- Add the sage and crumbled shell nuts to the pan for the last few minutes of cooking.
- Toast bread on a hot griddle pan, rub with cloves of garlic.
- Add the toast to the pan, taste, and adjust seasoning.

- Melt butter in a pan, add the mushrooms with chopped clove of garlic. Fry.
- Squeeze in a little lemon juice, blend until smooth.
- Boil salted water, add the spinach and cook until soft. Drain in a colander.
- Add remaining garlic to a frying pan with a splash of olive oil. Fry until golden.
- Add the pine nuts, sultanas and spinach and fry until warmed through.
- Season with salt and pepper and turn off the heat.
- Roll out the puff pastry on a sheet of baking parchment, then spread the mushroom mixture all over.
- In a large bowl, lightly toss together the spinach, squash and onion-bread mixture, then spoon it in a thick line down the middle of the pastry.
- Beat the egg with the milk and brush it over the pastry join to seal the join.
- Bake for 45 minutes until puffed up.

- Serve and enjoy.

Roasted chicken with mixed mushroom stuffing

Ingredients

- Olive oil
- 2 large handfuls of fresh white breadcrumbs
- 1 onion, peeled and finely chopped
- 1 free-range egg
- 4 cloves garlic, peeled and finely sliced
- 500g of mixed, interesting mushrooms
- 1 whole higher-welfare chicken
- Freshly ground black pepper
- 1 large handful of pine nuts
- 1 bunch of fresh thyme
- 1 lemon
- Sea salt

Directions

- Preheat your oven ready to 475°F.
- Heat olive oil in over a medium heat.
- Then, add onion together with the garlic, let cook for 10 minutes.
- Add the mushrooms with thyme leaves.

- Raise the heat to high, fry for 10 minutes.
- Remove, grate in the zest of the lemon and season.
- When the mixture has cooled, mix in the pine nuts and breadcrumbs.
- Add the egg. Push a quarter of the stuffing into pocket created in the chicken skin and roll the remaining mixture into balls and pop to one side.
- Cut your zested lemon in half and place in the chicken cavity with the remaining thyme sprigs.
- Place in a roasting tray, drizzle with olive oil and season with salt and pepper.
- Place in the oven. Cook for 40 minutes, then add mushroom stuffing balls to the tray.
- Continue to cook for 35 more minutes until golden.
- Serve and enjoy with fluffy roast potatoes and seasonal greens.

Creamy mushroom soup

Ingredients

- 1 onion
- Extra virgin olive oil
- 2 sticks of celery
- 6 slices of ciabatta
- 3 cloves of garlic
- Sprigs of fresh thyme
- 600g of mixed mushrooms
- 1.5 liters of organic chicken
- 75ml of single cream
- Sprigs of fresh flat-leaf parsley
- Olive oil

Directions

- Begin by heating a splash of olive oil in over a medium heat.
- Add the onion together with the celery, parsley stalks, garlic, thyme leaves, and mushrooms, cook until softened.
- Reserve 4 tablespoons of mushrooms.

- Boil the stock over a medium heat, lower the and simmer for 15 minutes.
- Season with sea salt and black pepper, then whisk until smooth.
- Pour in the cream, bring just back to the boil, then turn off the heat.
- Toast the ciabatta on a hot griddle pan, top with most of the reserved mushrooms
- Drizzle with extra virgin olive oil.
- Serve and enjoy with ciabatta crostini.

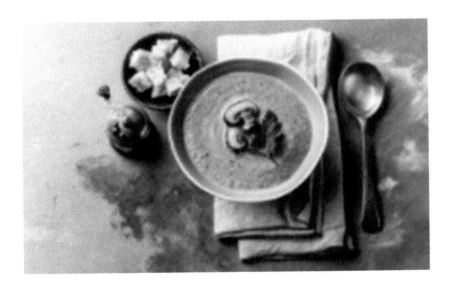

Italian style baked cheesy mushrooms

Ingredients

- 2 heads of dandelion
- 8 thin slices of ciabatta bread
- 2 handfuls of watercress
- 4 handfuls of mixed wild mushrooms
- Extra virgin olive oil
- Sea salt
- 2 handfuls of rocket
- Freshly ground black pepper
- 125g of scamorza
- ½ lemon
- 2 cloves of garlic
- 8 rashers smoked streaky bacon
- Sprigs fresh thyme
- 1 dried chili

Directions

- Preheat your oven to 350°F.
- Then, heat a griddle pan and toast the ciabatta slices until dark griddle marks.

- Tear up the toasted bread into chunks, toss with a drizzle of olive oil and a pinch of salt and pepper.
- In the same bowl, add the sliced garlic together with the chopped bacon and thyme leaves, torn mushrooms.
- Crumble in the dried chili, toss with your hands.
- Sprinkle the mixture fairly evenly on top of the bread, drizzle with olive oil, let bake for about 30 minutes, until the mushrooms are beginning to crisp up.
- Squeeze lemon juice into a jar. Top with extra virgin olive oil, and pinch of salt and pepper.
- Serve and enjoy.

Porchetta stuffed with wild mushrooms, celeriac mash and gravy

Ingredients

- 1 knob butter
- 2 bulbs garlic
- 2 lemons
- Sea salt
- A few slices stale bread
- 3 kg higher-welfare pork loin
- 500g of potatoes
- Olive oil
- 1 knob of butter
- 2 tablespoons fennel seeds
- 2 sticks celery
- 2 carrots
- 150ml of milk
- 1 small bunch fresh thyme
- 1 onion
- 1 small wineglass cider
- Freshly ground black pepper
- 1 large handful mixed wild mushrooms

- 1 tablespoon flour
- 565ml of organic chicken
- 1kg of celeriac

Directions

- Preheat your oven to high.
- Heat olive oil over a medium heat, add, the thyme leaves with mushrooms, garlic, and knob of butter. Fry for 10 minutes.
- Add the lemon zest with pinch of salt and pepper, let cool, and add the bread, toss.
- Lay the loin on a board, make a little pocket between the loin and the belly meat.
- Stuff the cooled mushroom mixture into the pocket.
- Season with salt and pepper.
- Place in the oven and immediately turn it down to 350°F. Rub up pestle fennel seeds and salt onto the skin. Let stay in the oven for 1 hour.
- Add the chopped vegetables and remaining bulb of garlic to the tray.
- Return to the oven to cook for another hour.

- Boil potatoes in salted water for 15 minutes.
- Drain and return to the pan with a knob of butter, seasoning and milk.
- Mash until smooth.
- Serve and enjoy.

Mushroom fish and chips style with posh vinegar

Ingredients

- 1 lemon
- 4 sprigs of fresh tarragon
- Freshly ground black pepper
- 2 sprigs of fresh thyme
- 4 handfuls of mixed mushrooms
- 6 white peppercorns
- 2 cloves garlic
- 400ml of white wine vinegar
- 1 small bunch fresh flat-leaf parsley
- 1 liter of olive oil
- 100g of plain flour
- Sea salt

Directions

- Put the whole sprigs of tarragon, thyme, peppercorns, and garlic slices into a bottle, topping with the vinegar.
- Let stay for hours.
- Heat olive oil over a medium heat.

- Combine flour with a generous pinch of salt and pepper, lemon zest on a large plate.
- Sprinkle mushrooms with a bit of water to moisten.
- Toss handfuls of the mushrooms in the seasoned flour to lightly coated.
- Deep-fry the mushrooms in batches until golden brown.
- Remove from the oil, drain any excess olive oil.
- Serve and enjoy with vinegar and parsley.

Chicken and mushroom pasta bake

Ingredients

- 150g of Parmesan cheese
- 20g of dried porcini mushrooms
- 200ml of white wine
- 300ml of single cream
- 320g of dried spaghetti
- Olive oil
- 4 higher-welfare chicken thighs
- Sea salt
- Freshly ground black pepper
- 2 cloves of garlic
- 1 sprig of fresh basil
- 350g of mixed fresh mushrooms

Directions

- Start by preheating your oven to 400°F.
- Heat a saucepan big enough to hold all the ingredients.
- Pour in a splash of olive oil.
- Season the chicken pieces with salt and pepper and brown them gently in the oil.

- Strain the porcini, reserving the soaking water.
- Add to the pan with the garlic and fresh mushrooms.
- Add the wine, with the strained porcini soaking water.
- Lower the heat down, let simmer until the chicken pieces are cooked through.
- Cook the spaghetti as directed on the package. Drain any excess water.
- Add the cream to the pan of chicken, then bring to the boil.
- Remove, season with salt and freshly ground black pepper.
- Add the drained spaghetti to the creamy chicken sauce and toss well.
- Add most of the Parmesan with basil, stir well.
- Transfer to an ovenproof baking dish, sprinkle with half the remaining cheese.
- Bake in the oven until golden brown.
- Serve and enjoy with sprinkle of zest cheese.

Baked mushrooms stuffed with ricotta

Baked mushroom stuffed with ricotta is an improved version of old classic featuring field mushrooms deliciously perfect for a Mediterranean Sea diet.

Ingredients

- Ricotta
- Lemon zest
- Chili
- Salt and pepper
- Oregano
- Parmesan
- Mushroom
- Rocket leaves

Directions

- Preheat your oven ready to 425°F.
- Place ricotta into a bowl with the lemon zest, chili, and bit of salt and pepper.
- Beat together, fold in chopped oregano with the Parmesan.
- Then, toss the mushroom caps in a little oil, salt and pepper.

- Lay them upside down on a baking tray to with small amounts of ricotta mixture.
- Spoon in the filling, sprinkle a little Parmesan over the top.
- Let bake in the preheated oven till golden in 15 minutes.
- Serve and enjoy sprinkled with some dressed rocket leaves.

Baked mushrooms

The baked mushrooms are baked in an earthly manner to elevated its deliciousness as expected of a Mediterranean Sea diet. It is flavored with natural garlic, onions, and herbs for a perfect Mediterranean sauce.

Ingredients

- 1 small bunch fresh flat-leaf parsley
- 8 large flat mushrooms
- Extra virgin olive oil
- 1 clove garlic
- 1 lemon
- Sprigs of fresh thyme
- 1 bunch of spring onions
- 250g of Taleggio cheese
- 2 thick slices bread
- 4 handfuls of rocket

Directions

- Preheat your oven ready to 400°F.
- Lay and sprinkle the mushrooms on a large baking tray with onions, garlic and thyme.
- Top with slices of Taleggio.

- Toss together the breadcrumbs with parsley sprinkled over the mushrooms.
- Let bake for 20 minutes in the preheated oven until breadcrumbs are brown.
- Dress the rocket with the lemon juice and some olive oil.
- Serve and enjoy with toasted ciabatta.

Lightning Source UK Ltd.
Milton Keynes UK
UKHW021228101022
410224UK00001B/16

9 781802 695946